ESSENTIAL GUIDE TO CELLULITIS

Comprehensive Insights for Diagnosis, Treatment, and Prevention

DR. CASEY LOREN

DISCLAIMER

This book's content is only meant to be used for general informative purposes. Although the author has taken great care to ensure the content is accurate and thorough, no warranties or assurances on the information's accuracy, correctness, or reliability are provided. It is recommended that readers employ their own judgment and discretion when applying any material found in this book to their particular situation.

The information in this book is not intended to replace professional advice, nor is the author an expert in any of the subjects covered. It is recommended that readers consult with experienced professionals regarding any particular issues or concerns.

Any name that may be mentioned or referred in this book does not imply endorsement, recommendation, or relationship on the part of the author with any person, entity, good, website, or association. These references are made only for informational purposes and are not meant to be taken as recommendations or endorsements.

The information contained in this book may cause readers to suffer loss or damage, for which the author disclaims all obligation and accountability. The only people accountable for the decisions and actions taken by readers using the information presented are themselves.

Any names, characters, companies, locations, activities, occasions, and incidents referenced in this book are either made up or the result of the author's imagination. Any likeness to real people, living or dead, or to real things is entirely coincidental.

This book's content may change at any time, without prior notice, according to the author.

The onus is on the reader to verify whether there have been any updates or revisions.

The reader accepts the conditions of this disclaimer by reading this book. Please do not read this book or use its contents if you do not agree to these terms.

Table of Contents

CHAPTER 1

COMPREHENDING CELLULITIS

An explanation and synopsis of cellulitis

A bacterial skin infection that targets the deeper tissue layers is called cellulitis. It usually happens when germs—most frequently Streptococcus or Staphylococcus—get into the skin through a crack or break, like a cut, wound, or insect bite. The affected area becomes heated, red, swollen, and inflamed as a result of this infection. Although cellulitis can affect any part of the body, it most frequently affects the feet and lower legs.

Motives and Risk Factors

Bacterial infections, typically caused by Streptococcus or Staphylococcus strains, are the main cause of cellulitis. The following are risk factors for contracting cellulitis:

1. Skin injuries: Bacteria can enter the body through cuts, abrasions, burns, surgical wounds, and insect bites.

2. Skin conditions: The skin barrier can be weakened by eczema, psoriasis, and athlete's foot, leaving the skin more vulnerable to infection.

3. Weakened immune system: Taking immunosuppressive medicines, having diabetes, HIV/AIDS, cancer, or other medical conditions can raise the risk.

4. Obesity: Being overweight can put a strain on the skin, causing fractures or cracks that allow germs to enter.

5. Lymphedema: The lymphatic system's capacity to combat infection may be compromised by limb swelling.

6. Age: Due to thinner skin and weakened immune responses, the elderly and young children are more susceptible.

Symptoms and Indications

Typical cellulitis symptoms and indicators include:

1. Warmth and redness in the impacted area

2. Inflammation and sensitivity

3. Soreness or pain

4. Stretched or taut skin

5. chills and a fever

6. Abscesses, blisters, or pus-filled lumps

7. enlarged lymph nodes close to the site of infection

Identification of Cellulitis

Based on a patient's medical history and physical examination, doctors can diagnose cellulitis. They might also carry out extra examinations, like:

1. Blood tests: To measure white blood cell counts and look for indications of infection.

2. Cultures: Gathering material from the afflicted region to pinpoint the precise bacteria that is causing the illness.

3. Imaging studies: To rule out more serious infections or consequences, X-rays, CT scans, or ultrasounds may be performed.

The Value of Early Identification

For cellulitis to be effectively treated and to avoid complications, early detection is essential.

Early diagnosis and intervention can help lower the chance of the infection spreading, resulting in a quicker recovery and better results.

Sorting Cellulitis Apart from Other Skin Disorders

Sometimes, cellulitis is confused with other skin disorders like:

1. Similar to bacterial skin illness, erysipelas usually affect the top layers of skin and have well-defined borders.

2. Necrotizing fasciitis: An uncommon but dangerous infection that spreads quickly and has the potential to kill tissue.

3. Dermatitis: Skin inflammation brought on by irritants or allergies, among other things.

4. Deep vein thrombosis: A blood clot in a deep vein that needs special care and may cause redness and edema.

Consequences Linked to Cellulitis

Cellulitis can result in problems like these if it is inadequately handled or left untreated:

1. Abscess formation: Within the diseased area, pus-filled pockets may form.

2. Bacteremia, or bloodstream infection, is a systemic infection caused by bacteria that enters the bloodstream.

3. Lymphangitis: An infection that affects the lymphatic vessels results in skin irritation and red splotches.

4. Recurrent or persistent bouts of cellulitis that need long-term care are referred to as chronic cellulitis.

Frequently Held Myths Regarding Cellulitis

Among the many myths surrounding cellulitis are the following:

1. It's always the result of bad hygiene: Although excellent hygiene practices can help prevent cellulitis, other risk factors can make the condition still happen.

2. It's a superficial skin infection: Unlike impetigo, which is also superficial, cellulitis affects deeper tissue layers.

3. Antibiotics are usually required; serious or systemic infections require antibiotics, but mild instances may heal with appropriate wound care and rest.

4. It's not serious: Untreated cellulitis, particularly in susceptible individuals, can result in significant complications.

Effects of Cellulitis on Day-to-Day Living

Many aspects of daily living can be significantly impacted by cellulitis, such as:

1. Pain and discomfort: The infection may interfere with every day activities by causing pain, soreness, and movement problems.

2. Emotional strain: Managing a persistent or reoccurring illness may cause worry, despair, or annoyance.

3. Financial costs: Paying for medical care, prescription drugs, and possible hospital stays can be expensive.

4. Lifestyle modifications: Patients might have to change their regular routines, such as

skipping certain activities or using compression clothing.

Treatment Trends for Cellulitis Today

Typically, cellulitis treatment entails:

1. Antibiotics: Depending on the infection's severity and bacterial cause, oral or injectable antibiotics may be recommended.

2. Wound care: To promote healing and stop subsequent infections, keep the injured area clean, dry, and elevated.

3. Pain management: For discomfort, over-the-counter or prescription painkillers may be advised.

4. Supportive measures: Adequate nutrition, rest, and hydration promote immune system health and general healing.

New developments in the management of cellulitis include:

1. Antibiotic stewardship: maximizing the use of antibiotics to minimize adverse effects and resistance.

2. Using cutting-edge treatments, dressings, and technologies to accelerate wound healing is known as advanced wound care.

3. Immunomodulatory agents: Studying treatments that strengthen the immune system to improve the body's ability to fight off infections.

4. Telemedicine and remote monitoring: extending alternatives for virtual follow-up visits and tracking the course of treatment.

CHAPTER 2

SKIN PHYSIOLOGY AND ANATOMY

Skin Structure

The biggest organ in the human body, the skin acts as a barrier to protect internal organs from the outside world. The epidermis, dermis, and hypodermis (subcutaneous tissue) are its three primary layers.

- **Epidermis:** Primarily composed of epithelial cells, this is the skin's outermost layer. Its primary job is to shield the body from outside influences like infections, UV rays, and dehydration.

Dermis: The dermis is the layer that lies beneath the epidermis and is home to a variety of anatomical features, including nerves, blood vessels, sweat glands, and hair follicles. It gives the skin elasticity and structural stability.

- **Hypodermis (Subcutaneous Tissue)**: Adipocytes, fat cells, and connective tissue make up this layer. It functions as an insulator, offering cushioning and assisting in controlling body temperature.

The Skin's Functions

The skin carries out several vital tasks:

1. **Protection:** It guards against dangers that are microbiological, chemical, and physical.

2. **Sensation:** Touch, pressure, pain, and temperature are all sensed by sensory receptors in the skin.

3. **Temperature Regulation:** The skin controls body temperature by producing sweat and dilatation and constriction of blood vessels.

4. **Synthesis of Vitamin D:** Sunlight exposure causes the skin to synthesize vitamin D, which is necessary for healthy bones.

5. **Immune Defence:** Immune cells in the skin protect the body from infections.

6. **Excretion:** Sweat glands are used to get rid of waste items.

Layers of the Skin

The epidermis, dermis, and hypodermis are the three main layers of skin, as was previously established. Every layer has unique properties and functions.

The Skin's Function in Immune Response

An important part of the body's immunological response is the skin. Specialized immune cells assist in identifying and eliminating infections that come into touch with the skin. Examples of these cells are immune cells in the dermis and Langerhans cells in the epidermis. Sebum and antimicrobial peptides produced by the skin are also antimicrobial.

The microbiota (microbial population) of the skin is diverse and has a role in the immune system and overall health. Cellulitis, a bacterial infection of the skin and underlying tissues, is one disorder that can result from specific causes upsetting this balance. Certain kinds of Streptococcus and Staphylococcus bacteria are frequently implicated in cellulitis.

Skin Changes and Ageing

The skin changes in several ways as we age. Among them are:

1. **Thinning of the Epidermis:** This may make a person more vulnerable to harm.

2. **Decreased Elastic Fibres and Collagen:** This causes wrinkles and a loss of skin suppleness.

3. **Slower Wound Healing:** Because of decreased collagen synthesis and cell turnover, aging skin heals more slowly.

Genetic Variations in Skin Conditions

Hereditary factors are important in defining the health of the skin and a person's vulnerability to specific disorders. For instance, certain people may be more susceptible to melanoma, psoriasis, and eczema due to genetic abnormalities. Comprehending these genetic variables is essential for tailored therapy and prophylactic measures.

Environmental Factors Affecting Skin Condition

Skin health can be impacted by environmental variables including pollution, UV radiation, and lifestyle decisions like smoking and eating habits. For example, skin cancer and early aging might result from UV exposure. To keep the skin healthy and beautiful, it must be shielded from environmental stresses.

Skin Care's Significance in Cellulitis Prevention

Preventing cellulitis requires good skin care routines that include frequent washing, moisturizing, and injury protection. Another way to lower the risk of bacterial infections is to treat cuts and wounds at once and to avoid spending a lot of time in damp settings.

Skin Disorders That Increase the Risk of Cellulitis

Cellulitis is more likely to develop in people with several skin diseases. Among them are:

1. **Eczema:** Eczema patients are more vulnerable to infections due to their compromised skin barrier.

2. **Diabetes:** Uncontrolled diabetes raises the risk of infections like cellulitis by compromising immune system performance and delaying wound healing.

3. **Peripheral Vascular Disease:** Infection and deterioration of the skin can result from decreased blood supply to the extremities.

4. **Immunocompromised States:** Immune system-compromising illnesses or therapies make people more vulnerable to infections, such as cellulitis.

Healthcare professionals can identify patients at increased risk for cellulitis and take appropriate preventive action by having a better understanding of these predisposing variables.

Healthcare practitioners can more effectively treat illnesses like cellulitis and advance general skin wellness by having a thorough understanding of the architecture and physiology of the skin, as well as its functions, immune response mechanisms, and factors impacting skin health.

CHAPTER 3

REASONS AND DANGER ELEMENTS

Cellulitis Caused by Bacteria:

germs are the main cause of cellulitis, and Streptococcus and Staphylococcus germs are the most frequent offenders. Insect bites, wounds, and even fissures in dry skin are examples of breaches or cuts where these germs might infiltrate the skin. Staphylococcus aureus and Group A Streptococcus are especially noteworthy since they are commonly linked to cellulitis infections. Bacterial cellulitis must be treated quickly to stop it from invading deeper into the skin or leading to more serious side effects, such as bloodstream infections.

Viral causes of cellulitis are less frequent than bacterial ones. But other viruses, such as varicella-zoster virus (VZV) and herpes simplex virus (HSV), can cause skin infections that mimic cellulitis. These viral infections might resemble cellulitis symptoms by causing skin inflammation and redness. Since treatment strategies for bacterial and viral infections range greatly, accurate diagnosis is crucial.

Candida and other dermatophytes are examples of the fungal organisms that cause fungal cellulitis, sometimes referred to as dermatophytic cellulitis. These fungi can infect the skin, particularly in warm, humid settings. Fungal cellulitis shares many of the same symptoms as bacterial cellulitis, including redness, swelling, and itching. Nonetheless, antifungal drugs are required to treat fungal cellulitis, emphasizing the significance of a precise diagnosis.

Cellulitis's Pathogenic Causes:

Additionally, certain worms, ticks, and mites can cause cellulitis. For example, bacteria can enter the skin from a tick bite and cause cellulitis. There may be a higher prevalence of parasitic illnesses in some geographical areas or among people who work outside. The risk of parasitic cellulitis can be decreased with appropriate preventive measures, such as wearing protective clothing and insect repellents.

Medical Disorders Increasing the Risk of Cellulitis:

The chance of getting cellulitis might be raised by several underlying medical issues. These include venous insufficiency, diabetes, lymphedema, peripheral vascular disease, and chronic skin disorders like psoriasis and eczema. Individuals suffering from these ailments frequently have weakened skin barriers or inadequate immunological responses, which increases their vulnerability to cellulitis. Effectively treating these illnesses is crucial to avoiding recurrent bouts of cellulitis.

Immune System Deficiencies and the Risk of Cellulitis:

Cellulitis is more common in people with compromised immune systems, such as cancer patients, HIV/AIDS patients, and organ transplant recipients on immunosuppressive medications. They are more susceptible to bacterial, viral, fungal, and even opportunistic infections that might result in cellulitis because of their weakened immune system. Preventing cellulitis and other severe infections requires vigilant immune status management together with close observation.

Cellulitis-Related Lifestyle Factors:

The risk of cellulitis might be increased by specific lifestyle choices. Skin infections and cellulitis are more common as a result of poor hygiene habits, such as sharing personal objects that can harbor bacteria or improperly cleansing wounds. Furthermore, bad behaviors like smoking and binge drinking can impair immunity, leaving people more vulnerable to diseases like cellulitis.

Occupational Cellulitis Risks:

Cellulitis risk is increased in occupations including construction, farming, and healthcare that need regular exposure to environmental risks. Skin injuries and subsequent cellulitis can result from contact with soil, polluted water, sharp objects, or infectious organisms in hospital environments. Using the right safety equipment, following safety procedures, and taking timely care of wounds are critical to lowering the incidence of occupational cellulitis.

Recurrent Cellulitis: Factors to Consider and Handling:

Some people have recurrent bouts of cellulitis, which is frequently brought on by underlying conditions such as lymphatic blockage, chronic venous insufficiency, or recurrent skin infections. Managing recurrent cellulitis requires identifying and treating these underlying causes. To stop recurrence, long-term preventive interventions may be required. These may include skin care regimens, compression therapy for venous insufficiency, and, in some situations, prophylactic antibiotics.

Cellulitis Prevention Techniques:

A variety of tactics are used to prevent cellulitis, such as taking good care of wounds, practicing good hygiene, avoiding skin injuries, dressing in protective clothing in high-risk situations, effectively managing underlying medical conditions, and getting the necessary vaccinations, such as the tetanus vaccine. Reducing the prevalence of cellulitis and enhancing general skin health need educating people about these preventive actions and encouraging proactive healthcare behaviors.

CHAPTER 4

PRESENTATION OF CLINICAL DATA AND DIAGNOSIS

Common Cellulitis Symptoms

Localized skin redness, warmth, swelling, and soreness are common signs of cellulitis. Additionally, the afflicted area may feel tight or hard to the touch. As the infection worsens, symptoms could include chills, fever, exhaustion, and in extreme situations, the formation of skin blisters or ulcers.

Unusual Cellulitis Presentations

Discolored patches of skin without the usual warmth and swelling are examples of atypical presentations of cellulitis. Cellulitis can occasionally afflict odd places including the face, genitalia, or the perineum. Atypical symptoms might also appear in patients with weakened immune systems or long-term medical disorders.

Differential Cellulitis Diagnosis

Differential diagnoses including deep vein thrombosis, contact dermatitis, insect bites, erysipelas, necrotizing fasciitis, and other skin infections should be taken into account while evaluating a patient with suspected cellulitis. For an appropriate diagnosis, a complete clinical evaluation and analysis of the patient's medical history are essential.

The Value of a Physical Exam

The physical examination is essential for the diagnosis of cellulitis. Medical professionals examine the afflicted area for indications of inflammation, such as warmth, redness, swelling, and discomfort. The assessment of the patient's general health, vital signs, and any concomitant symptoms aids in identifying the extent of the infection and directs the course of treatment.

Cellulitis Laboratory Tests

A complete blood count (CBC), which measures raised white blood cell count (an indicator of infection), erythrocyte sedimentation rate (ESR), and C-reactive protein (CRP) levels—markers of inflammation—are commonly used in laboratory testing for cellulitis. If a systemic infection is suspected, blood cultures may be taken.

Imaging Research in the Diagnosis of Cellulitis

Imaging tests like ultrasounds, CT scans, or MRIs could be suggested to check for problems like the development of an abscess or deep tissue involvement, or in situations where the diagnosis is unclear. Planning a course of treatment can be aided by these investigations' ability to visualize the degree of tissue inflammation.

Sensitivity testing and cultures

To determine the bacterium causing the infection and inform the choice of antibiotic, cultures can be taken from the afflicted skin region or any drainage. To support targeted therapy and prevent antibiotic resistance, sensitivity testing is used to identify the antibiotics that work best against the identified bacteria.

Cellulitis Biopsy Procedures

A skin biopsy may be necessary in some circumstances to rule out other skin disorders that mimic cellulitis or to determine whether there is deeper tissue involvement. Under a microscope, biopsy samples are inspected to check for particular histological alterations that are indicative of cellulitis.

Chronic Cellulitis and Its Difficulties to Diagnose

Because of its recurrent bouts and symptoms that can be confused with those of other skin disorders, chronic cellulitis presents diagnostic complications. It is necessary to take into account differential diagnoses such as lymphedema, venous insufficiency, and inflammatory skin conditions. The main goals of long-term treatment techniques include finding the root causes and averting flare-ups.

Diagnostic Standards and Recommendations

The clinical presentation, physical examination results, and supporting laboratory or imaging data serve as the basis for the cellulitis diagnosis criteria. Guidelines for the diagnosis and treatment of cellulitis are available from groups like the Infectious Diseases Society of America (IDSA), with an emphasis on the significance of precise assessment and suitable antibiotic therapy.

Healthcare professionals can accurately diagnose cellulitis, distinguish it from related disorders, and use focused treatment plans to enhance patient outcomes by attending to each of these factors thoroughly.

CHAPTER 5

METHODS OF THERAPY
Cellulitis Treatment Using Antibiotics

Overview: The mainstay of treatment for cellulitis is the use of antibiotics, which work to eradicate bacterial infections and stop them from spreading. Macrolides, cephalosporins, and penicillins are among the antibiotics that are frequently administered.

Justification: Antibiotics, such as Streptococcus or Staphylococcus species, target the underlying bacterial cause. They are selected taking into account the patient's allergies, the level of infection, and patterns of local antibiotic resistance.

Administration: Usually administered intravenously for serious infections necessitating hospitalization, orally for minor instances. Though it varies, it usually lasts five to fourteen days.

Supervision: Consistent evaluation of antibiotic response, including a decrease in inflammation, redness, and pain. If early therapy is unsuccessful, cultures may dictate modifications to treatment plans.

Topical Cellulitis Treatments

Usage: Topical antibiotics, such as mupirocin, can be used in conjunction with systemic therapy to treat localized infections or mild cases of cellulitis.

Application: Apply directly to skin areas that are impacted, avoiding open wounds and mucous membranes. Topical application should come first with wound cleansing and good hygiene.

Benefits include a more focused effect, a decrease in systemic adverse effects, and the possibility of managing moderate instances without hospitalization.

Adjunctive Treatments: Antidepressants, steroids, etc.

Steroids: Occasionally used as an adjuvant to lessen inflammation, particularly when there is a lot of discomfort or swelling. It's critical to closely watch for side effects including immunosuppression.

NSAIDs: Reduce inflammation and provide pain relief. Patients with gastrointestinal problems or renal impairment should use caution.

Analgesics: Reduce symptoms and improve patient comfort while cellulitis is being treated.

Clotting and Wound Maintenance

Guidelines: Prioritise wound hygiene, manage moisture and prevent further infections. Simple gauze dressings to sophisticated hydrocolloid or foam dressings are examples of dressings.

 Wound Cleaning: Use saline or antiseptic solutions regularly to clean wounds; stay away from harsh chemicals as these could impede recovery.

Moisture Balance: To encourage the growth of granulation tissue and avoid excessive dryness or exudate buildup, maintain ideal moisture levels.

Dressing Selection: based on the size, depth, and quantity of exudate from the wound. The best possible wound healing is ensured by routine evaluation and dressing changes.

Surgical Procedures for Serious Instances

Indications: Surgery may be required in cases with severe cellulitis with abscess formation, necrotizing fasciitis, or poor response to medicinal therapy.

Procedures: Incision and drainage of abscesses; fasciotomy in compartment syndrome instances; debridement of necrotic tissue.

After Operation: Vigilant observation to promote wound closure, manage infection, and restore function. Following surgery, antibiotic medication may continue.

Handling Complicated Situations

Systemic Complications: Keep an eye out for fever, tachycardia, hypotension, and altered mental status, which are all indicators of sepsis. It is essential to intervene quickly and use broad-spectrum antibiotics together with fluid resuscitation.

Chronic Cellulitis: To avoid recurring outbreaks, treat underlying risk factors such as lymphedema or venous insufficiency.

Follow-Up: Frequent clinic visits guarantee that the cellulitis resolves, watch for complications, and modify treatment as necessary.

Self-Care and Patient Education

Main Takeaways: Inform patients on wound maintenance, using antibiotics as prescribed, recurrence warning indicators, and prophylactic steps.

Self-Monitoring: Train patients to spot early warning indicators of worsening cellulitis, like a rise in discomfort, swelling, or redness.

Preventive Measures: Place a strong emphasis on wound care, skin hygiene, preventing skin damage, and controlling underlying illnesses that raise the risk of cellulitis.

New Treatments and
Scientific Developments

Phage Therapy: The experimental application of bacteriophages to target particular strains of bacteria, potentially providing a different approach to treatment.

Immunomodulators: New studies investigate how immunotherapy can strengthen the host's defenses against infections that cause cellulitis.

Genetic Studies: In the future, tailored treatment strategies may be informed by knowledge of genetic susceptibilities to cellulitis.

Comprehensive Methods for Treating Cellulitis

Complementary Therapies: To enhance general healing and immunological function, take into consideration the adjunctive use of complementary techniques such as acupuncture, herbal medicines, or nutritional supplements.

Collaborative Care: Arrange for the safe and efficient integration of therapies by working with practitioners of complementary medicine.

Customising Care to Meet Patient Needs

Individualised Approach: When creating treatment regimens, take into account patient characteristics such as age, comorbidities, allergy history, and social support.

Incorporate patients in treatment conversations, taking into account their preferences, worries, and expectations through **Shared Decision-Making**.

Multidisciplinary Team: Cooperation between medical professionals—such as chemists, wound care nurses, and specialists in infectious diseases—improves the quality and efficiency of treatment.

With an emphasis on a holistic strategy to address infection, promote wound healing, minimize complications, and empower patients in their recovery path, every facet of cellulitis treatment is essential for comprehensive patient management.

CHAPTER 6

DIFFICULTIES AND OUTLOOK

Localised Cellulitis Complications

Even while cellulitis is frequently successfully treated, there may be several local problems. Among them are:

1. **Abscess Formation**: Pus-filled pockets that need to be drained may form inside the damaged tissue.

2. **Necrotizing Fasciitis**: This uncommon but serious consequence causes tissue loss quickly and necessitates surgery right away.

3. **Chronic Cellulitis**: Recurrent or chronic episodes of cellulitis can cause long-term skin

changes and possibly harm to the lymphatic system in certain individuals.

Sepsis and Systemic Complications

Sepsis and systemic problems can result from severe cases of cellulitis. Among them are:

1. **Sepsis**: A potentially fatal illness in which organ failure results from the body's reaction to an infection.

2. **Septic Shock**: Severe sepsis can result in organ failure and dangerously low blood pressure.

3. **Spread of Infection**: If the infection gets into the bloodstream, it can damage several organs and cause meningitis or endocarditis, among other consequences.

Recurrent Cellulitis: Preventative Measures and Risk Factors

The following are risk factors for recurrent cellulitis:

1. **Lymphedema**: Cellulitis risk is increased by chronic swelling brought on by injury to the lymphatic system.

2. **Skin Conditions**: Wounds, dermatitis, and eczema may serve as harbors for germs.

3. **Immunosuppression**: Immune system-depressing illnesses or drugs make people more vulnerable.

Among the preventative techniques are:

1. **Skin Care**: Maintaining the skin's cleanliness, hydration, and barrier against damage.

2. **Compression Therapy**: Compression clothing can help people with lymphedema feel less swollen.

3. **Prophylactic Antibiotics**: To avoid recurrences, it is occasionally necessary to prescribe long-term antibiotics.

Cellulitis's Effect on Life Quality

Quality of life can be considerably impacted by cellulitis by:

1. **Discomfort and Pain**: Acute symptoms including swelling, redness, and pain can be upsetting.

2. **Functional Limitations**: Mobility and day-to-day activities may be restricted in severe situations.

3. **Emotional Toll**: Social isolation, anxiety, and depression can result from recurring or chronic cellulitis.

Long-Term Outlook and Continued Care

The degree of the infection, any underlying medical issues, and how well the patient responds to treatment are some of the variables that affect the long-term prognosis for cellulitis. The following care could consist of:

1. **Monitoring**: Consistent evaluations to look for problems or recurrence.

2. **Education**: Teaching patients how to take care of their skin, avoid getting infections, and spot cellulitis early on.

3. **Referral to experts**: Dermatologists or infectious disease experts may need to be consulted in cases of complicated cellulitis or recurrent cases.

Adverse Effects of Insufficient or Delayed Medical Care

Inadequate or delayed cellulitis therapy can result in:

1. **Persistent Infection**: Chronic cellulitis may result from an infection that may not fully go away.

2. **Spreading Infection**: Abscesses or systemic infection can result from bacteria that go to deeper tissues.

3. **Resistant Infections**: Treatment may become more difficult when bacteria become resistant to antibiotics over time.

Chronic Cellulitis's Psychological Effects

Psychological consequences associated with chronic cellulitis include:

1. **Anxiety**: Worries about chronic infections or lasting effects.

2. **Depression**: Changes in appearance, functional restrictions, and ongoing discomfort can all lead to depression.

3. **Physique Image Issues**: Skin abnormalities or scars can impact one's perception of their physique and self-worth.

Functional Recovery and Rehabilitation

The goals of cellulitis rehabilitation are:

1. **Physical Therapy**: To restore function, strength, and movement.

2. **Occupational Therapy**: Supporting everyday life activities and adaptable techniques.

3. **Psychological Support**: Group therapy or counselling to deal with emotional difficulties.

Complication Predictive Factors

Among the variables that could indicate cellulitis complications are:

1. **Underlying Health Conditions**: Immunosuppression, diabetes, and peripheral vascular disease raise the risk.

2. **Infection Severity**: Significant cellulitis, abscesses, or systemic signs suggest a higher risk.

3. **Prior Episodes**: Complications may be more likely in those with recurrent cellulitis.

Techniques for Handling Difficult Cases

Handling complex cases of cellulitis entails:

1. **Multidisciplinary Approach**: Including experts in wound care, surgery, and infectious disease medicine.

2. **Advanced Imaging**: To determine the degree of tissue involvement, an MRI or CT scan may be required.

3. **Surgical Intervention**: For lymphatic system rebuilding, debridement of necrotic tissue, or abscess drainage.

Healthcare professionals can improve patient outcomes and quality of life by effectively assessing, treating, and preventing complications by having a thorough awareness of various elements of cellulitis.

CHAPTER 7

PREVENTIVE TECHNIQUES

The Value of Good Skin Care

Cellulitis must be avoided by practicing proper skin cleanliness. Frequent washing of the skin with gentle soap and water helps to eliminate dirt and bacteria, which lowers the chance of infection. It is crucial to keep hands, legs, and feet clean and dry as these are areas that are vulnerable to cellulitis. Maintaining neat nails, refraining from sharing personal goods like towels or razors, and washing your hands well are other aspects of proper hygiene.

First Aid and Wound Care

To avoid cellulitis, wounds must be properly and promptly cared for. Before covering any cuts, scratches, or wounds with a sterile bandage, clean them with soap and water and apply an antibiotic or antiseptic ointment. It's important to keep an eye out for infection symptoms in wounds, such as redness, swelling, warmth, or pus, and to get medical help if any appear.

Identifying Early Infection Symptoms

Preventing the progression of cellulitis requires the identification of the early indicators of infection. At the location of an injury or wound, symptoms could include redness, swelling, warmth, soreness, and pain. Additional symptoms including chills, fever, and exhaustion could also point to an infection. Treating these symptoms as soon as possible will stop problems and infections from spreading.

Immunisation and Vaccination

Certain forms of cellulitis, such as those brought on by germs like Streptococcus and Staphylococcus, can be significantly avoided by vaccination. Immunizations against wounds or traumas, such as the tetanus vaccine, can lower the incidence of cellulitis. Furthermore, maintaining current vaccination records by medical professionals' recommendations is critical to general health and immune system performance.

Lifestyle Changes to Prevent Cellulitis

There are lifestyle changes that can lower the risk of cellulitis. Immune system stimulation and general well-being can be achieved by eating a balanced diet high in vitamins and nutrients, staying physically active, and maintaining a healthy weight. Reducing alcohol intake and tobacco usage also strengthens the immune system and improves general health.

Precautions in High-Risk Situations

It is imperative to take extra precautions to prevent cellulitis in high-risk environments, such as hospitals or unsanitary regions. These could include adhering to infection control procedures, using the correct personal protective equipment (PPE), such as masks and gloves, and maintaining good hygiene and sanitation practices.

Healthcare Professionals' Role in Prevention

By providing knowledge, early infection diagnosis, and treatment, healthcare providers are essential in the prevention of cellulitis. They oversee patients for indications of infection, offer advice on wound care, vaccinations, and hygiene habits, and move quickly to intervene when necessary.

Education and Public Health Initiatives

Campaigns for education and public health bring cellulitis prevention techniques to the attention of local populations. These programs could consist of outreach campaigns, workshops, and educational materials that stress the value of wound care, vaccination, and good hygiene in lowering the prevalence of cellulitis.

Interventions Based on the Community

To execute preventive measures, community organizations, individuals, and healthcare practitioners collaborate in community-based initiatives. These interventions could involve setting up health fairs, giving immunization clinics, offering resources for wound care, and encouraging the community to adopt healthy lifestyles.

Long-term cellulitis prevention requires integrating preventive techniques into everyday activities. This entails following appropriate hygiene procedures, routinely monitoring for any indications of infection, maintaining current vaccination records, and embracing a healthy lifestyle. Developing a habit of prevention lowers the incidence of cellulitis and enhances general health.

The prevalence of cellulitis can be considerably decreased, improving health outcomes for both individuals and communities, by incorporating these preventive techniques into daily life and raising awareness at both the individual and community levels.

CHAPTER 8

HAVING CELLULITIS AND GETTING BY

Patient and Carer Coping Techniques:

Cellulitis requires a combination of physical self-care and psychological toughness to handle. Patients must carefully follow their doctor's instructions, keep the affected region clean and elevated, and frequently check for any indications that their symptoms are getting worse. In addition, practicing stress-reduction strategies like deep breathing, meditation, or taking up a hobby can assist in controlling any anxiety or frustration related to the illness. Essential functions for carers include helping with everyday tasks, offering emotional support, and promoting adherence to treatment programs.

Resources and Support Networks:

Resources and Support Networks:

Patients with cellulitis and those who care for them can gain a lot by attending support groups and consulting with medical experts who specialize in wound care or infectious diseases. These communities provide insightful information, emotional support, and helpful tips for properly managing cellulitis. Online resources can also connect people with pertinent resources and offer up-to-date information. Examples of these resources include credible medical websites and forums that are moderated by healthcare professionals.

Dietary Guidelines for the Management of Cellulitis:

There is no one "cellulitis diet," but eating a healthy, balanced diet is essential for promoting both general health and immunological function. If you want to encourage healing and lower inflammation, concentrate on eating an abundance of fruits, vegetables, lean proteins, and whole grains. Stable blood sugar levels and immune system support can also be achieved by avoiding processed foods and excessive sugar.

Physical Activity and Exercise Guidelines:

Patients with cellulitis may benefit from moderate exercise, adapted to their capacities, as it improves circulation and general health. But it's imperative to stay away from activities that could strain or injure the afflicted area. Getting advice from a physical therapist or healthcare professional can assist create an exercise program that is both safe and efficient.

Psychological Effects and Assistance for Mental Health:

Stress, anxiety, or sadness can be brought on by having cellulitis, which can hurt the mental health of both patients and carers. Mental well-being can be considerably enhanced by seeking assistance from mental health specialists, taking part in counseling or therapy sessions, and engaging in self-care practices like mindfulness or relaxation exercises.

Coordination of Social and Work Activities:

It takes careful preparation and communication to manage cellulitis while juggling work obligations and social engagements. Open communication about the illness with coworkers, employers, and social networks can promote acceptance and support. During times of active treatment or recuperation, it could be required to make adjustments or modifications to work schedules.

Cellulitis Patients' Travel Considerations:

Patients with cellulitis should speak with their doctors before departing to make sure they have enough medication on hand and are aware of any safety measures or suggestions. When traveling, it's critical to follow proper hygiene procedures, drink enough water, and shield the afflicted region from potential infection sources.

Fighting for Patients' Rights:

Effective management of cellulitis requires enabling people to speak out for their rights, obtain high-quality medical care, and seek treatment as soon as possible. The whole experience of receiving care can be improved by being aware of and standing up for patient rights, such as timely access to medical records, informed consent, and courteous treatment.

Family and Carers' Role:

In addition to providing practical help with everyday duties, family members and carers are essential in helping patients with cellulitis feel supported and have their needs met by the hospital system. A comprehensive approach to care involves collaboration with healthcare providers, effective communication, and education about the problem.

Success Stories: Living Well Despite Cellulitis:

Telling the success stories of those who have successfully treated their cellulitis and seen improvements in their condition might give people hope and encouragement. These accounts demonstrate the value of tenacity, following prescribed courses of action, and receiving support from loved ones and medical professionals in overcoming the difficulties associated with cellulitis.

CHAPTER 9

NEW DEVELOPMENTS IN THE EPIDEMIOLOGY OF CELLULITIS

The epidemiology of cellulitis, an infection of the skin and subcutaneous tissue, has changed over time. These patterns include shifts in the incidence rates, the demographics affected, the role of comorbidities and environmental variables, and the emergence of new causal pathogen strains. To enable focused preventative efforts and optimal clinical therapy, research in this field aims to uncover trends, risk factors, and variations in cellulitis presentation among various groups and geographic regions.

Technological Progress in Diagnostics

From traditional clinical assessment to the use of cutting-edge technologies like imaging modalities (MRI, ultrasound), laboratory tests (cultures, biomarkers), and digital health tools (telemedicine, mobile apps for monitoring), the field of cellulitis diagnosis has seen tremendous advancements. These developments are intended to increase the precision of cellulitis diagnosis, distinguish it from disorders that resemble it, direct the selection of the most suitable course of therapy, and promote overall patient outcomes using prompt and targeted interventions.

Innovative Therapeutic Strategies

The discipline of managing cellulitis is still investigating new therapy strategies outside of traditional antibiotics. This covers the creation of novel wound care techniques, immunomodulators, topical medications, and targeted antimicrobial approaches such as antimicrobial peptides or bacteriophage therapy. To ensure effective therapy while minimizing side effects and increasing patient recovery, research also focuses on improving already recommended antibiotic regimens, investigating combination medicines, and addressing antibiotic resistance challenges.

Precision Medicine and Genomic Research

Determining the genetic foundation of host-pathogen interactions, treatment response variability, and cellulitis susceptibility is largely dependent on genomic investigations. This makes it possible to apply the concepts of precision medicine, making it possible to conduct personalized risk assessments, custom therapeutic actions based on genetic profiles, and forecast treatment outcomes. The development of tailored therapeutics, optimal antibiotic stewardship, and personalized patient care are all facilitated by the use of genetics in cellulitis research.

Development of Vaccines to Prevent Cellulitis

A growing number of studies are being conducted to create a vaccination to prevent cellulitis, with a focus on important bacterial pathogens such as Streptococcus pyogenes and Staphylococcus aureus. The main areas of research are antigenic target identification, vaccine formulations (e.g., polysaccharide conjugates, protein-based), immunization tactics (including their possible application in high-risk populations), and assessments of the safety, effectiveness, and long-term protection of vaccines. Immunizations have the potential to lessen the incidence of cellulitis, stop recurrent infections, and address the issue of antibiotic resistance.

Issues with Global Health and Cellulitis

Due to variables like socioeconomic inequality, impediments to healthcare access, regional differences in pathogen incidence, and climate-related effects on skin infections, cellulitis poses serious global health concerns. To tackle these issues, research endeavors aim to establish fairness in the prevention, diagnosis, and treatment of cellulitis, promote global cooperation, and customize interventions for various healthcare environments while taking into account the cultural, economic, and environmental factors that influence health.

Collaborative Research Projects

To improve patient care and our understanding of cellulitis, collaborative research projects are essential. Multidisciplinary teams made up of physicians, researchers, public health specialists, business associates, patient advocates, and legislators are involved in these initiatives. Partnerships make it easier to share data, standardize procedures, conduct large-scale epidemiological studies, conduct clinical trials for cutting-edge solutions, and conduct implementation research to close the gap between the creation of knowledge and the delivery of healthcare.

Priorities for Patient-Centered Research

Understanding patient experiences, preferences, treatment outcomes, and the effects on quality of life are given top priority in patient-centered research on cellulitis. This includes using patient views in study design, intervention development, and healthcare policy formulation; it also entails using shared decision-making processes, patient-reported outcome measures, and qualitative investigations. Research has greater significance, responsiveness, and alignment with addressing the actual needs and priorities of cellulitis patients when patient perspectives are included.

Ethical Issues in Research on Cellulitis

Research integrity, responsible sharing of findings, informed consent, privacy protection, fair access to interventions, and research integrity are all critical ethical considerations in medical research. The ethical values of beneficence, non-maleficence, justice, autonomy, and respect for participant rights are upheld by ethical frameworks, which also serve as guidelines for research conduct. To preserve integrity, trust, and ethical norms in cellulitis research projects, ethical reflection and supervision are essential.

Integrating Clinical Practice with Research

Improving cellulitis treatment and patient outcomes requires putting research results into clinical practice. Evidence synthesis, guideline formulation, provider education programs, new intervention implementation techniques, and quality improvement measures in healthcare delivery are all part of this translation. To ensure that evidence-based methods are successfully incorporated into normal clinical care and improve outcomes for cellulitis patients, it is necessary to bridge the gap between research and practice through collaboration between researchers, clinicians, patients, legislators, and healthcare systems.

Each of these fields reflects a dynamic and changing field of study on cellulitis, emphasizing interdisciplinary efforts to further understanding, enhance patient care, and address the wider public health consequences of this prevalent infectious disease.

CHAPTER 10

FUTURE PROSPECTS FOR RESEARCH

Present Developments in the Study of Cellulitis

Currently, cellulitis research is concentrated in a few important areas. Investigating the microbiome's function in the onset and recurrence of cellulitis is one trend. Researchers are also looking into how antibiotic resistance affects the course of treatment for cellulitis. Furthermore, research is being done to learn more about the inflammatory processes connected to cellulitis and how to target them for more potent treatments.

New and Emerging Therapies

Several novel treatments are being investigated for the treatment of cellulitis. These include immunomodulatory drugs to control the inflammatory response, innovative antibiotic formulations with increased activity against resistant bacteria, and therapies that destroy biofilms to increase the penetration and effectiveness of antibiotics.

Advances in Trauma Care

Advanced dressings that encourage wound healing and lower the risk of infection are among the innovations in wound care for patients with cellulitis. To enhance outcomes in situations of severe cellulitis, technologies including bioengineered skin substitutes and negative pressure wound therapy are also being used.

Development of Vaccines

While there isn't a vaccination specifically for cellulitis, efforts are being made to create ones that target the germs that cause the illness, like Streptococcus pyogenes and Staphylococcus aureus. For susceptible people, particularly those who have a history of infections, these vaccinations may be able to avoid bouts of cellulitis.

Progress in Diagnostic Methods

Cellulitis diagnostic methods are changing as a result of the emergence of imaging modalities like MRI and ultrasound to evaluate deeper tissue involvement. Additionally, molecular diagnostic techniques are being developed to quickly determine the microorganisms causing the problem and direct the proper use of antibiotics.

Research Focused on the Patient

The goal of cellulitis patient-centered research is to enhance treatment compliance and quality of life. This covers research on self-management techniques, patient education, and psychosocial therapies to deal with the psychological effects of recurrent bouts of cellulitis.

Cooperation Projects

Partnerships involving patient advocacy organizations, researchers, industry stakeholders, and healthcare practitioners are a part of collaborative efforts. These partnerships make it easier to share data, conduct clinical trials, and put best practices for managing cellulitis into practice.

Perspectives on Global Health

With variations in incidence, causal microorganisms, and therapeutic accessibility internationally, cellulitis is a global health concern. To combat resistance, research on global health emphasizes the need to address disparities in cellulitis care, particularly in places with limited resources, and to promote antimicrobial stewardship.

Difficulties in the Management of Cellulitis

Antibiotic resistance, recurrent infections, delayed therapy due to misdiagnosis, and consequences like lymphedema and abscess formation are among the difficulties in managing cellulitis. Two continuous issues are optimizing antimicrobial therapy and coordinating interdisciplinary care.

Possibilities to Enhance Patient Results

Early diagnosis and treatment of cellulitis, individualized antibiotic regimens based on microbiological data, telemedicine integration for follow-up care, and patient education on preventive measures including wound care and cleanliness are all opportunities to improve patient outcomes in the management of cellulitis.

We can further our understanding of cellulitis, better treatment approaches, and ultimately improve outcomes for patients suffering from this illness by tackling these research areas and future directions thoroughly.